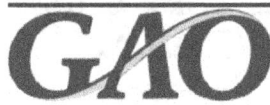

United States Government Accountability Office

Testimony
Before the Subcommittee on Workforce
Protections, Committee on Education
and the Workforce, U.S. House of
Representatives

For Release on Delivery
Expected at 10 a.m. EDT
Wednesday, July 10, 2013

FEDERAL EMPLOYEES' COMPENSATION ACT

Analysis of Benefits Under Proposed Program Changes

Statement of Andrew Sherrill, Director,
Education Work Force and Income Security

July 10, 2013

GAO Highlights

Highlights of GAO-13-730T, a testimony before the Subcommittee on Workforce Protections, Committee on Education and the Workforce, U.S. House of Representatives

FEDERAL EMPLOYEES' COMPENSATION ACT

Analysis of Benefits Under Proposed Program Changes

Why GAO Did This Study

In 2012, the FECA program provided more than $2.1 billion in wage-loss compensation to federal workers who sustained injuries or illnesses while performing federal duties. Total-disability beneficiaries with an eligible dependent are compensated at 75 percent of gross wages at the time of injury and those without are compensated at 66-2/3 percent. Benefits are adjusted for inflation and are not taxed nor subject to age restrictions. Some policymakers have raised questions about the level of FECA benefits, especially compared to federal retirement benefits. Proposals to revise FECA for future total- and partial- disability beneficiaries include: setting initial FECA benefits at a single rate (66-2/3 or 70 percent of applicable wages at time of injury), regardless of whether the beneficiary has eligible dependents; and converting FECA benefits to 50 percent of applicable wages at time of injury—adjusted for inflation—once beneficiaries reach full Social Security retirement age.

This testimony presents results of GAO's four recent reports on FECA issues. It summarizes (1) potential effects of the proposals to compensate total-disability FECA beneficiaries at a single rate; (2) potential effects of the proposal to reduce FECA benefits to 50 percent of applicable wages at full Social Security retirement age for total-disability beneficiaries; and (3) how partial disability beneficiaries might fare under the proposed changes. To do this work, GAO conducted simulations comparing FECA benefits to income (take-home pay or retirement benefits) a beneficiary would have had absent an injury, and conducted seven case studies of partial disability beneficiaries.

View GAO-13-730T. For more information, contact Andrew Sherrill at (202) 512-7215 or sherrilla@gao.gov

What GAO Found

GAO's simulation found that under the current Federal Employees' Compensation Act (FECA) program, the median wage replacement rate—the percentage of take-home pay replaced by FECA—for total-disability beneficiaries was 88 percent for U.S. Postal Service (USPS) beneficiaries and 80 percent for non-USPS beneficiaries in 2010. GAO also found that proposals to set initial FECA benefits at a single compensation rate would reduce these replacement rates by 3 to 4 percentage points under the 70-percent option and 7 to 8 percentage points under the 66-2/3 percent option. Beneficiaries with dependents would receive reduced FECA benefits under both options. The decreases in wage replacement rates were due to the greater proportion of beneficiaries who had a dependent—over 70 percent of both USPS and non-USPS beneficiaries.

In GAO's simulation comparing FECA benefits to retirement benefits, GAO found that under the current FECA program, the median FECA benefit package for total-disability retirement-age beneficiaries was 37 and 32 percent greater than the median 2010 retirement benefit package for USPS and non-USPS beneficiaries, respectively. This analysis focused on individuals covered under the Federal Employees Retirement System (FERS), which generally covers employees first hired in 1984 or later, and covered about 85 percent of the federal workforce in 2009. GAO also found that the proposal to reduce FECA benefits at the full Social Security retirement age would result in a median FECA package roughly equal to the median FERS retirement package in 2010. However, the median years of service for the FERS annuitants GAO analyzed was about 16 to 18 years, so these simulations did not capture a fully mature retirement system and likely understated the future FERS benefit level. Consequently, GAO also simulated a mature FERS system—intended to reflect future benefits of workers with 30-year careers—and found that the median FECA benefit package under the proposed change would be from 22 to 35 percent less than the median FERS retirement package.

Partial-disability beneficiaries are fundamentally different from total-disability beneficiaries, as they receive reduced FECA benefits based on a determination of their earning capacity. GAO's seven case studies of partial-disability beneficiaries showed that how they might fare under the proposed FECA changes can vary considerably based on their individual circumstances, such as their earning capacity and actual levels of earnings. For example, among GAO's case studies, those beneficiaries with high earning capacities may elect to retire under FERS and would likely not be affected by the proposed FECA reduction at retirement age because their potential retirement benefits were substantially higher than their current or proposed reduced FECA benefit levels. In contrast, those beneficiaries with low earning capacities had potential retirement benefits that were lower than their current FECA benefits and the proposed FECA reduction at retirement age would reduce their FECA benefits.

Chairman Walberg, Ranking Member Courtney and Members of the Subcommittee:

I am pleased to be here today to discuss our work on proposed changes to benefit levels in the Federal Employees' Compensation Act (FECA) program. We recently issued three reports on how proposed changes would affect FECA beneficiaries covered under the Federal Employees Retirement System (FERS) and a prior report that examined the characteristics and income of FECA beneficiaries in comparison to retired annuitants under the Civil Service Retirement System (CSRS).[1]

In 2010, the FECA program paid $1.9 billion in cash benefits to federal workers who sustained injuries or illnesses while performing federal duties.[2] The U.S. Department of Labor (Labor) administers FECA and bases FECA benefits on an employee's wages at the time of injury and whether the employee has eligible dependents. In addition, consideration is given to the beneficiary's ability to work after the injury. Specifically, beneficiaries unable to return to work—total-disability beneficiaries—who have an eligible dependent are compensated at 75 percent of gross wages at the time of injury and those without an eligible dependent are compensated at 66-2/3 percent.[3] These benefits are adjusted for inflation and are not taxed nor subject to age restrictions. Some policymakers have raised questions about the level of FECA benefits, especially compared to the retirement benefits under FERS, which generally covers

---

[1]GAO, *Federal Employees' Compensation Act: Effects of Proposed Changes on Partial-disability Beneficiaries Depend on Employment After Injury*, GAO-13-143R (Washington, D.C.: December 7, 2012), GAO, *Federal Employees' Compensation Act: Analysis of Proposed Changes on USPS Beneficiaries*, GAO-13-142R (Washington, D.C.: November 26, 2012), GAO, *Federal Employees' Compensation Act: Analysis of Proposed Program Changes*, GAO-13-108 (Washington, D.C.: October 26, 2012), and GAO, *Federal Employees' Compensation Act: Benefits for Retirement-Age Beneficiaries*, GAO-12-309R (Washington, D.C.: February 6, 2012).

[2]The receipt of FECA benefits is generally the exclusive remedy for being injured on the job and a federal employee is prohibited from recovering damages for such injury under another statute.

[3]Beneficiaries who are determined to have some wage earning capacity—partial-disability beneficiaries—are compensated based on the difference between wages at the time of injury and wages that Labor determines they are able to earn in a suitable job. Those with a dependent are compensated at 75 percent of this difference and those without an eligible dependent at 66-2/3 percent of the difference.

employees first hired in 1984 or later. As of September 30, 2009, about 85 percent of the federal workforce was covered by FERS.

Proposals to revise FECA include the following changes to the benefits for future total and partial-disability beneficiaries:[4]

- Set initial FECA benefits at a single rate (either 66-2/3 or 70 percent of applicable wages at time of injury), regardless of whether the beneficiary has eligible dependents.

- Convert FECA benefits to 50 percent of applicable wages at time of injury—adjusted for inflation—once beneficiaries reach the full Social Security retirement age.

My statement today will focus on our findings regarding (1) the potential effects of the proposals to compensate total-disability FECA beneficiaries at a single rate regardless of having dependents; (2) the potential effects of the proposal to reduce FECA benefits for total-disability beneficiaries to 50 percent of applicable wages at Social Security retirement age; and (3) how partial-disability beneficiaries might fare under the proposed changes. This statement is drawn primarily from our four prior reports analyzing the effects of proposed changes to FECA.

To consider the effect of compensating total-disability FECA beneficiaries at the single rate of either 66-2/3 or 70 percent, we conducted simulations that compared the extent to which FECA and the proposed revision would replace a FECA beneficiary's take-home pay by analyzing a set of federal employees who had never been injured and who were employed at the end of fiscal year 2010. [5] We used a matching methodology, which allows us to capture the counterfactual of having never been injured and use it to

---

[4]The proposals analyzed are Labor's "Federal Injured Employees' Reemployment Act of 2010" technical assistance discussion draft, January 13, 2011 and S. 1789, 112th Cong., tit. III (2012). Both proposals include setting initial FECA benefits at a single rate—Labor proposed 70 percent and S. 1789 proposed 66-2/3 percent. Both proposals would reduce benefits at full Social Security retirement age to 50 percent of applicable wages.

[5]We defined take-home pay as gross wages reduced by mandatory retirement contributions and federal and state income taxes (assuming a single dependent) and did not take discretionary deductions into account. The analyses were based on snapshots in 2010 and did not consider any cumulative effects of the proposed FECA revisions on lifetime income.

benchmark the adequacy of benefits. [6] We conducted separate simulations for non-USPS and USPS beneficiaries because their data were organized differently in separate databases and the USPS FECA population is substantial—43 percent of FECA beneficiaries in 2010 were employed by USPS at the time of injury. Once we matched the FECA beneficiaries to the relevant set of federal workers, we calculated their hypothetical FECA and hypothetical revised FECA benefits, and projected these initial benefits to 2010.[7] We calculated the proportion of 2010 take-home pay replaced by the simulated FECA benefit, or wage replacement rate.[8]

---

[6]We matched recent total disability FECA beneficiaries to these employees in order to ensure the two groups of individuals were similar. Our matches were based on work-related characteristics—such as employing agency and blue collar versus white collar classification. We also included personal characteristics that may be important in terms of career and wage growth, such as the date and age when the employees started their federal careers, as well as their wage histories prior to the injury. For more details on the similarity of the matched set of FECA beneficiaries and federal employees, see appendix II of GAO-13-108 (non-USPS) and enclosure I of GAO-13-142R (USPS).

[7]After matching, we focus solely on the federal worker—rather than the FECA beneficiary—because doing so is more precise than comparing the benefit of the FECA beneficiary to the earnings of the matched federal worker. By considering only the federal worker, we are able to capture the wage replacement rate, the proportion of take-home pay replaced by FECA, in a way that meaningfully accounts for career growth while avoiding undue imprecision in wage replacement rates that could be attributed to salary differences between the federal worker and the matched FECA beneficiary. We calculated initial benefits to reflect the timing of the corresponding FECA beneficiary's injury.

[8]At the time of injury, wage replacement rates are actually greater than FECA compensation rates. For example, given a dependent and gross wages of $50,000, the FECA benefit is $37,500 (75 percent). Assuming 15 percent taxes, take home pay would be $42,500, and the wage replacement rate would be 88 percent (37,500/42,500). Policymakers can target wage replacement rates; however, there is no consensus on the appropriate wage replacement rate for workers' compensation programs, such as FECA. Such decisions involve balancing the goals of benefit adequacy and incentives to return to work. In 1972, the National Commission on State Workmen's Compensation Laws endorsed a move towards 80 percent of spendable pay or take-home pay. A 1998 GAO report on FECA also cited this 80 percent benchmark; see GAO, *Federal Employees' Compensation Act: Percentages of Take-Home Pay Replaced by Compensation Benefits*, GAO/GGD-98-174 (Washington, D.C.: August 1998). In 2004, a report by the National Academy of Social Insurance used two-thirds of gross wages as a target replacement rate for workers' compensation programs. See H. Allan Hunt, editor, *Adequacy of Earnings Replacement in Workers' Compensation Programs, A Report of the Study Panel on Benefit Adequacy of the NASI Workers' Compensation Steering Committee* (Washington D.C.: 2004).

By using 2010 take-home pay, we factored in missed career growth into the wage replacement rates we calculated. Although FECA was not designed to compensate for missed career growth, we used a matching methodology that allowed us to measure the adequacy of benefits with respect to the counterfactual. Specifically, we captured the extent to which FECA beneficiaries are able to maintain the standard of living they would have had absent an injury.[9]

To compare FERS to total-disability FECA benefits, we also relied on a matching technique,[10] and conducted our analysis for both the current FECA program and the proposal to reduce benefits at full retirement age.[11] We projected simulated FECA benefits to 2010 and compared these FECA benefits, supplemented by a Thrift Savings Plan (TSP) annuity, to the actual FERS benefit packages.[12] The FERS benefit package includes the FERS annuity, Social Security benefits, and TSP

---

[9]Alternatively, one could use a method that does not account for missed career growth. For instance, in our 1998 FECA report (GAO/GGD-98-174), we calculated wage replacement rates by comparing FECA benefits to take-home pay at the time of injury, adjusted for inflation. That approach measured the degree to which beneficiaries were able to maintain the standard of living they would have had at the time of injury. We took that approach in part because of the data available at the time of the report, GAO/GGD-98-174. The report found that, on average, FECA benefits replaced over 95 percent of wages at the time of injury for beneficiaries, including both USPS and non-USPS beneficiaries. In its comments on our 1998 report, Labor took issue with the fact that we did not take account of missed promotions. Labor stated that it is almost certain that some percentage of injured workers would have received promotions, thus lowering the wage replacement rate. The availability of additional data and the improved methods employed in our recent analysis allow us to present an assessment of the adequacy of benefits that includes career growth. For additional discussion of the merits of accounting for missed career growth in assessing the adequacy of benefits, see Hunt, 2004.

[10]For details on the match and subsequent analysis, see appendix II of GAO-13-108 enclosure I of GAO-13-142R.

[11]This approach captures retirement benefits in the counterfactual case of having never been injured and is consistent with our February 2012 FECA report, which compared FECA benefits to retirement benefits under the Civil Service Retirement System. See GAO, *Federal Employees' Compensation Act: Benefits for Retirement-Age Beneficiaries* GAO-12-309R (Washington, D.C.: February 6, 2012).

[12]FECA beneficiaries cannot receive FECA benefits concurrently with the FERS annuity. Further, Social Security benefits attributable to federal service are offset by FECA after retirement.

annuities. [13] However, FERS had only been in place 26 years in 2010, so we did not capture a fully mature system. [14] To capture future FECA beneficiaries, we conducted another simulation to account for a mature FERS. In this simulation, we examined the effects of missing part of a 30-year career due to injury. [15]

To determine the effects on partial-disability beneficiaries, we used different methods to analyze how they might fare under proposed FECA revisions. We did not conduct the types of simulations we used for total-disability beneficiaries, in part because Labor does not keep data about their total income (including any earnings) in an electronic database. Instead, we reviewed partial-disability beneficiary case files to examine how their post-injury employment outcomes varied (e.g., re-employed by the federal government, re-employed in the private sector, or unemployed) and changed over time and judgmentally selected 7 beneficiaries to present as case studies. [16] The results from these case studies are not generalizable to all partial-disability beneficiaries.

The work on which this testimony was based was conducted in accordance with generally accepted government auditing standards. Those standards require that we plan and perform the audit to obtain

[13]To conduct our simulations, we used data from the 2010 Integrated Federal Employees' Compensation System (iFECS); 1988- 2010 data from the Central Personnel Data Files (CPDF); 1995-2010 data from USPS Human Capital Enterprise System (HCES); 2010 FERS annuitant data; 2000-2012 Thrift Savings Plan (TSP) data; and Social Security benefit data from the Master Beneficiary Record (MBR). We determined that the data we used were sufficiently reliable for the purposes of the reports.

[14]By mature FERS, we mean a retirement system in place at least 30 years to give a full range of income levels and investment growth. Federal employees age 62 with over 30 years of service accrue retirement benefits at a slightly higher rate. In addition, having 4 additional years of TSP contributions and growth can lead to greater account balances. Our current data has limited observations on FERS annuitants with more than 25 years of service. Without taking account of the mature system, we understate the future FERS benefit.

[15]We then simulated different scenarios by varying the percentage an individual contributed to the TSP and the rate of growth for TSP balances. Please see appendix II of GAO-13-108 for more details about our simulation of a mature FERS.

[16]We selected the 7 case studies to show variation in wage earning capacity and post-injury job outcomes, including 4 beneficiaries who returned to work (2 to federal service and 2 to private sector jobs) and whose wage earning capacity was based on their actual wages, and 3 beneficiaries whose wage earning capacity was based on a Labor estimate of what the beneficiary could earn in an appropriate job placement.

sufficient, appropriate evidence to provide a reasonable basis for our findings and conclusions based on our audit objectives. We believe that the evidence obtained provides a reasonable basis for our findings and conclusions based on our audit objectives.

Background

FECA

FECA provides cash benefits to eligible federal employees who suffer temporary or permanent disabilities resulting from work-related injuries or diseases. Labor's Division of Federal Employees' Compensation in the Office of Workers' Compensation Programs (OWCP) administers the FECA program and charges agencies for whom injured employees worked for benefits provided. These agencies subsequently reimburse Labor's Employees' Compensation Fund from their next annual appropriation. FECA benefits are adjusted annually for cost-of-living increases[17] and are neither subject to age restrictions nor taxed. USPS has large FECA program costs. At the time of their injury, 43 percent of FECA beneficiaries in 2010 were employed by USPS, as shown in table 1.

Table 1: Number of FECA Beneficiaries per Agency in 2010

Agency	All FECA beneficiaries	
	Number	Percentage
USPS	130,483	43
Department of Veterans Affairs	26,157	9
Department of Homeland Security	25,408	8
Navy	19,919	6
Army	19,852	6
Air Force	12,728	4
Department of Justice	11,001	4
Department of Agriculture	10,691	3
Department of the Interior	9,205	3
Defense agencies[a]	6,101	2

[17]FECA and Social Security are adjusted by the same price index (CPI-W).

Agency	All FECA beneficiaries	
	Number	Percentage
Other agencies[b]	35,360	12
Total	**306,905**	**100**

Source: GAO analysis of Labor data.

[a]Defense Agencies covered include the Defense Contract Audit Agency, Defense Logistics Agency, and the Defense Contract Management Agency, among others.

[b]The remaining agencies listed each have less than 2 percent of the total number of beneficiaries receiving workers' compensation benefits, and fewer than 5,275 beneficiaries each.

One way to measure the adequacy of FECA benefits is to consider wage replacement rates, which are the proportion of pre-injury wages that are replaced by FECA. Wage replacement rates that do not account for missed career growth capture the degree to which a beneficiary is able to maintain his or her pre-injury standard of living whereas wage replacement rates that account for missed career growth capture the degree to which a beneficiary is able to maintain his or her foregone standard of living (i.e., standard of living absent an injury). Data limitations can preclude calculating wage replacement rates that account for missed career growth; however, doing so provides a more complete story of the comparison between an injured worker and his or her counter-factual of having never been injured. Wage replacement rates can be targeted by policy-makers; however, there is no consensus on what wage replacement rate policies should target.[18]

FECA and Retirement under FERS

FECA beneficiaries receive different benefits past retirement age than workers who retire under a federal retirement system. Specifically, under FERS, federal retirees have a benefit package comprised of three components: the FERS annuity, which is based on years of service; the TSP, which is similar to a 401(k); and Social Security benefits.[19] FECA benefits do not change at retirement age and beneficiaries cannot receive a FERS annuity and FECA benefits simultaneously. In addition, FECA

---

[18]H. Allan Hunt, editor, *Adequacy of Earnings Replacement in Workers' Compensation Programs, a Report of the Study Panel on Benefit Adequacy of the NASI Workers' Compensation Steering Committee* (Washington, D.C.: 2004).

[19]FERS, which generally covers employees first hired in 1984 or later, replaced the Civil Service Retirement System (CSRS). According to OPM, about 80 percent of federal annuitants that were on OPM's rolls in 2011 were CSRS annuitants. Among those CSRS annuitants, the average years of federal service was almost 30 years.

beneficiaries cannot contribute to their TSP accounts post-injury, but they can receive benefits accrued from contributions made to their TSP accounts prior to being injured. In addition, Social Security benefits attributable to federal service are offset by FECA.

Partial and Total-disability

If an individual has an extended disability and no current capacity to work, OWCP determines that he or she is a total-disability beneficiary and calculates long-term FECA benefits as a proportion of the beneficiary's entire income at the time of injury.[20] In 2010, 31,880 FECA beneficiaries received long-term total-disability cash benefits.[21]

Alternatively, if an individual recovers sufficiently to return to work in some capacity, OWCP determines that he or she is a partial-disability beneficiary and reduces his or her FECA benefits from the total-disability amount. For such partial-disability beneficiaries, OWCP calculates long-term benefits based on any loss of wage earning capacity (LWEC), as compared to their pre-injury wages.[22] A beneficiary's LWEC may be based on the difference between their pre-injury wages and their actual post-injury earnings if the beneficiary has found employment that OWCP determines to be commensurate with their rehabilitation. Alternatively, OWCP constructs a beneficiary's LWEC based on the difference between pre-injury wages and OWCP's estimate of what the FECA beneficiary could earn in an appropriate job placement (constructed earnings). In 2010, 10,594 FECA beneficiaries received long-term partial-disability cash benefits.[23]

---

[20]The amount of time a beneficiary receives these long-term total-disability benefits varies depending on the extent and speed of recovery.

[21]See GAO, *Federal Employees' Compensation Act: Benefits for Retirement-Age Beneficiaries*, GAO-12-309R (Washington, D.C.: February 6, 2012) for more information on the number and types of FECA beneficiaries in 2010. In this report we found that, compared to their federal CSRS retired counterparts, non-USPS long-term, full-time FECA beneficiaries typically received higher benefits in 2010. The median annual FECA benefit of $35,614 was about 26 percent higher than the median annual annuity received by retirees, which was $28,289, after adjusting for the effects of taxes.

[22]We use the term "pre-injury wages" for clarity. OWCP calculates long-term benefits based on the current pay rate—at the time of this calculation—of the job the beneficiary held at the time of injury.

[23]See GAO-12-309R for more information on the number and types of FECA beneficiaries in 2010.

FECA Operations	In addition to our work on FECA benefit levels, we have also conducted work on program integrity and management. We have identified several weaknesses in these areas.[24] Most recently, in April 2013, we found examples of improper payments and indicators of potential fraud in the FECA program, which could be attributed, in part, to oversight and data-access issues. We also found that FECA program requirements allow claimants to receive earnings, and earnings increases, without necessarily resulting in adjustment of FECA compensation. We recommended that the Secretary of Labor assess the feasibility of developing a cost-effective mechanism to share FECA compensation information with states. Labor agreed with the recommendation and stated that it will undertake a review to determine whether such data sharing and reporting is feasible.
Proposed FECA Revisions Would Reduce Median Wage Replacement Rates and Increase the Difference between Total-Disability Beneficiaries With and Without a Dependent	Our simulations of the effects of compensating non-USPS and USPS total-disability beneficiaries at the single rate (regardless of the presence of dependents) of either 66-2/3 or 70 percent of wages at injury, reduced the median wage replacement rates. Median wage replacement rates overall, and within the subgroups we examined, were generally lower under the 66-2/3 percent compensation proposal.

---

[24]GAO, *Federal Employees' Compensation Act: Case Examples Illustrate Vulnerabilities That Could Result in Improper Payments or Overlapping Benefits,* GAO-13-386 (Washington, D.C.: April 3, 2013). GAO, *Federal Employees' Compensation Act: Status of Previously Identified Management Challenges,* GAO-12-508R (Washington, D.C.: March 21, 2012). GAO, *Federal Employees' Compensation Act: Preliminary Observations on Fraud-Prevention Controls,* GAO-12-402 (Washington, D.C.: January 25, 2012). GAO, *Federal Employees' Compensation Act: Preliminary Observations on Fraud-Prevention Controls,* GAO-12-212T (Washington, D.C.: November 9, 2011). GAO, *Federal Employees' Compensation: Better Data and Management Strategies Would Strengthen Efforts to Prevent and Address Improper Payments,* GAO-08-284 (Washington, D.C.: February 26, 2008).

Proposed Single Rates Would Reduce Wage Replacement Rates

Compared to the current FECA program, both proposals reduced 2010 median wage replacement rates for total-disability non-USPS and USPS beneficiaries, as shown in figure 1. The decreases in the overall median wage replacement rates were due to the greater proportion of beneficiaries who had a dependent—73 percent of non-USPS beneficiaries and 71 percent of USPS beneficiaries. Beneficiaries with a dependent received lower compensation under both proposals whereas beneficiaries without a dependent saw their compensation increase or stay the same.

Figure 1: 2010 Wage Replacement Rates under FECA and the Proposed Revisions

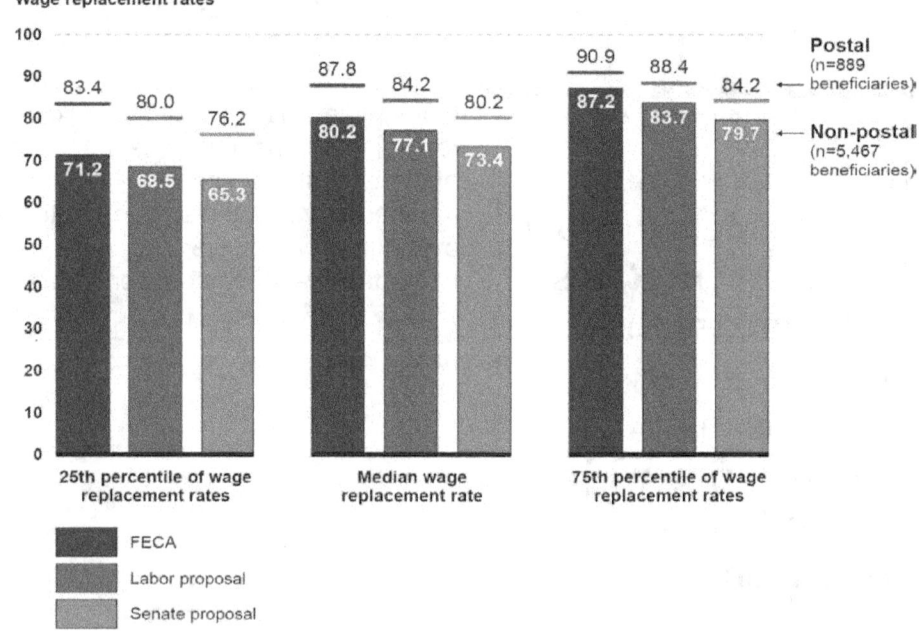

Source: GAO analysis of simulation results.

Note: Wage replacement rates are calculated based on 2010 take-home pay and account for missed income growth. Postal refers to USPS and non-postal refers to non-USPS.

As shown in the middle group of bars in figure 1, the results of our simulation indicate that median wage replacement rates for USPS beneficiaries were generally higher than those for non-USPS beneficiaries. In both cases, the wage replacement rates account for missed income growth, as they are simulated based on 2010 take-home pay. All else equal, FECA beneficiaries who would have experienced more income growth—from the time of injury through 2010—had lower wage replacement rates than did those beneficiaries who would have experienced less income growth absent their injury. In general, USPS beneficiaries missed less income growth due to their injury than did non-USPS beneficiaries. Consequentially, USPS beneficiaries had higher wage replacement rates than non-USPS beneficiaries. For example, 4 out of 5 USPS beneficiaries in our analysis would have had less than 10 percent income growth had they never been injured. In contrast, 2 out of 5 non-USPS beneficiaries would have had less than 10 percent income growth, absent an injury.

Under our simulations, both proposals increased the difference in wage replacement rates between beneficiaries with and without a dependent, increasing the magnitude and reversing the direction of the difference in median wage replacement rates, as shown in figure 2. Had we been able to account for the actual number of dependents, beneficiaries with dependents would have had lower wage replacement rates and thus the difference between median wage replacement rates would have been smaller under FECA and larger under both proposals.[25]

---

[25] Our data did not include information on the number of dependents, so we assumed a single dependent. All else equal, having more dependents would generally increase take-home pay (because of smaller tax liabilities) and therefore result in lower wage replacement rates. For more information, see GAO-13-108.

Figure 2: 2010 Median Wage Replacement Rates for Beneficiaries With and Without a Dependent

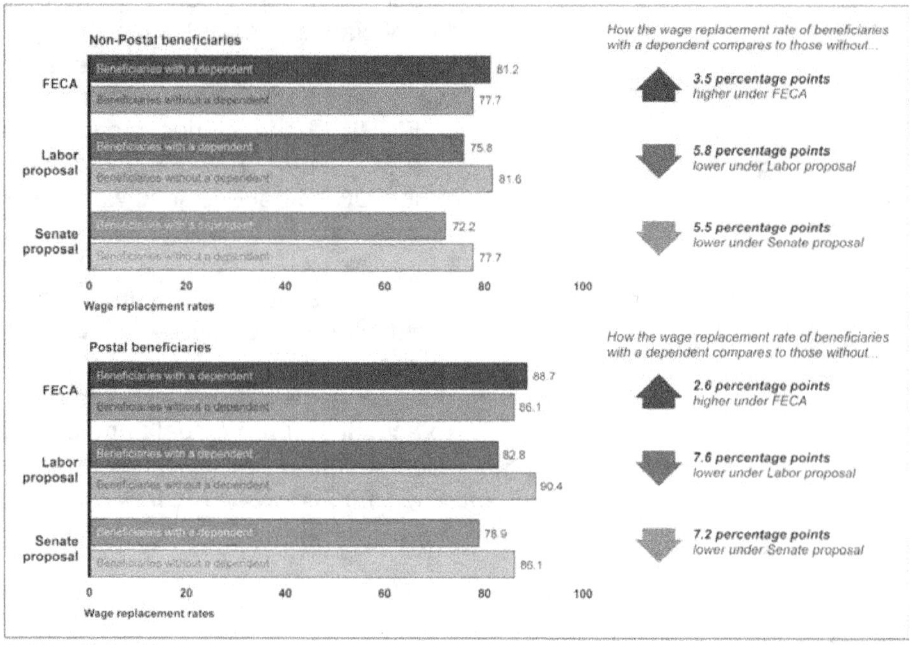

Non-Postal beneficiaries

How the wage replacement rate of beneficiaries with a dependent compares to those without...

FECA
- Beneficiaries with a dependent: 81.2
- Beneficiaries without a dependent: 77.7
- 3.5 percentage points higher under FECA

Labor proposal
- Beneficiaries with a dependent: 75.8
- Beneficiaries without a dependent: 81.6
- 5.8 percentage points lower under Labor proposal

Senate proposal
- Beneficiaries with a dependent: 72.2
- Beneficiaries without a dependent: 77.7
- 5.5 percentage points lower under Senate proposal

Wage replacement rates

Postal beneficiaries

How the wage replacement rate of beneficiaries with a dependent compares to those without...

FECA
- Beneficiaries with a dependent: 88.7
- Beneficiaries without a dependent: 86.1
- 2.6 percentage points higher under FECA

Labor proposal
- Beneficiaries with a dependent: 82.8
- Beneficiaries without a dependent: 90.4
- 7.6 percentage points lower under Labor proposal

Senate proposal
- Beneficiaries with a dependent: 78.9
- Beneficiaries without a dependent: 86.1
- 7.2 percentage points lower under Senate proposal

Wage replacement rates

Source: GAO analysis of simulation results.

Note: Wage replacement rates are calculated based on 2010 take-home pay and account for missed income growth. Postal refers to USPS and non-postal refers to non-USPS.

For other beneficiary subgroups we examined, the proposals did not reduce wage replacement rates disproportionately to the reduction in the overall median.[26] However, we found that under current FECA policy and both proposals, wage replacement rates for some beneficiaries, such as those who, due to injury earlier in their careers, missed out on substantial income growth, were substantially lower than the overall median. FECA was not designed to account for missed income growth and thus total-disability beneficiaries who missed substantial income growth had lower wage replacement rates—outweighing the cumulative effect of FECA's annual cost of living adjustments—as shown in figure 3.

---

[26]We examined subgroups of beneficiaries by state tax rates, General Schedule (GS) level at injury and GS level growth (non-USPS), and income percentile category at injury (USPS). The GS classification and pay system covers the majority of civilian white-collar Federal employees.

Figure 3: 2010 Median Wage Replacement Rates by Missed Income Growth

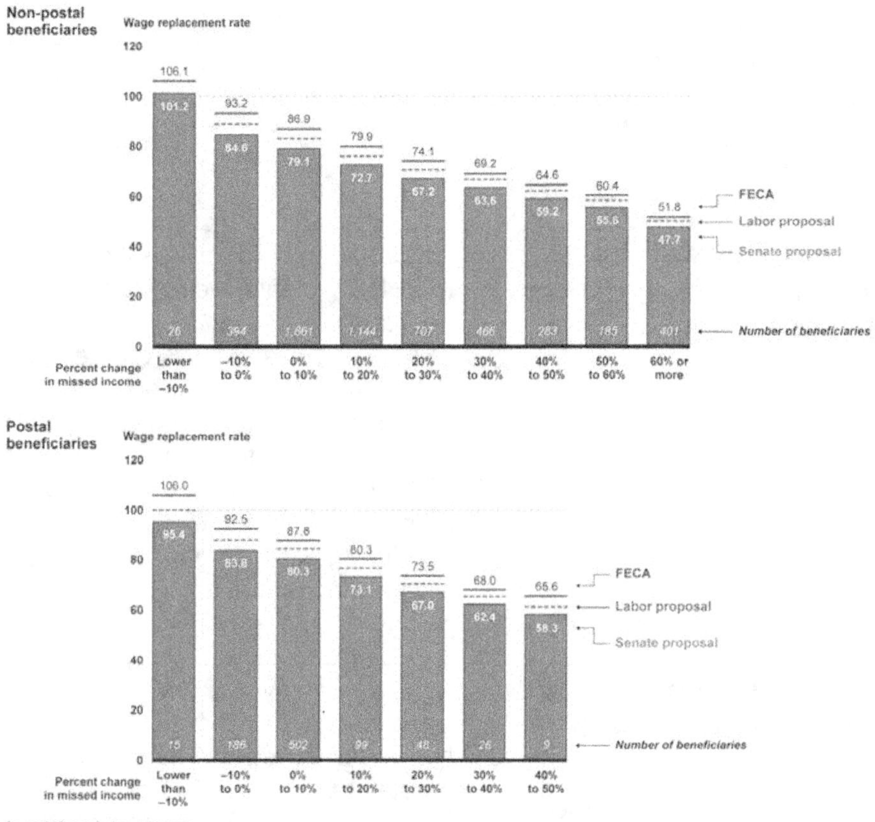

Non-postal beneficiaries

Wage replacement rate

Percent change in missed income	Lower than −10%	−10% to 0%	0% to 10%	10% to 20%	20% to 30%	30% to 40%	40% to 50%	50% to 60%	60% or more
FECA	106.1	93.2	86.9	79.9	74.1	69.2	64.6	60.4	51.8
Labor proposal	101.2	84.6	79.1	72.7	67.2	63.6	59.2	55.6	47.7
Number of beneficiaries	26	394	1,861	1,144	707	466	283	165	401

Postal beneficiaries

Wage replacement rate

Percent change in missed income	Lower than −10%	−10% to 0%	0% to 10%	10% to 20%	20% to 30%	30% to 40%	40% to 50%
FECA	106.0	92.5	87.8	80.3	73.5	68.0	65.6
Labor/Senate proposal	95.4	83.8	80.3	73.1	67.0	62.4	58.3
Number of beneficiaries	15	186	502	99	48	26	9

Source: GAO analysis of simulation results

Note: Intervals do not include the upper endpoints. In addition, not enough USPS beneficiaries had missed income growth over 50% to report their wage replacement rates. Wage replacement rates are calculated based on 2010 take-home pay and account for missed income growth. Postal refers to USPS and non-postal refers to non-USPS.

Years of Service Play a Key Role in the Comparison between FECA and FERS Benefits

Current Median FECA Benefit Packages Exceed 2010 FERS Benefit Packages

According to our retirement simulation comparing current FECA benefits to FERS benefits, we found that the overall median FECA benefit package (FECA benefits and TSP annuity) for both USPS and non-USPS FECA beneficiaries was greater than the current median FERS retirement benefit package (FERS annuity, TSP annuity, and Social Security). Specifically, the median FECA benefit package for non-USPS beneficiaries was 32 percent greater than the current median FERS—and 37 percent greater for USPS FECA beneficiaries.[27] This implies that in retirement, FECA beneficiaries generally had greater income from FECA and their TSP in comparison to the FERS benefits they would have received absent an injury.

Increased Years of Service Were Associated with Increased FERS Benefits Relative to FECA Benefits for 2010 Annuitants

Although the overall median FECA benefit was substantially higher than the median FERS benefit for 2010 annuitants, the difference between the two varies based on years of service. Our simulations showed that median FECA benefit packages were consistently greater than median FERS benefit packages across varying years of service; however, the gap between the two benefits narrowed as years of service increased. This occurred in large part because FERS benefits increase substantially with additional years of service. For example, under our simulation non-USPS beneficiaries whose total federal career would have spanned less than 10 years had a median FECA benefit that was about 46 percent greater than the corresponding FERS benefit. In contrast, non-USPS beneficiaries whose total federal career would have spanned 25-29 years had a median FECA benefit that was 16 percent greater than the corresponding FERS benefit. For USPS beneficiaries, those whose total federal career would have spanned less than 10 years had a median

---

[27] In our datasets, non-USPS FERS annuitants had a median of about 16 years of service, while USPS annuitants had a median of 18 years.

FECA benefit that was about 65 percent greater than the corresponding FERS benefit, while beneficiaries whose total federal career would have spanned between 20 and 24 years had a median FECA benefit that was 23 percent greater than the corresponding FERS benefit.

Proposals would Roughly Equalize FECA and FERS Benefit Packages for 2010 Annuitants

Based on our simulation, we found that reducing FECA benefits once beneficiaries reach retirement age to 50 percent of wages at the time of injury would result in an overall median for the reduced FECA benefit package (reduced FECA plus the TSP) that was about 6 percent less than the median FERS benefit package for non-USPS annuitants. Under our simulation, for USPS annuitants, the reduced FECA benefit package would be approximately equal to the median 2010 FERS benefit package. This implies that under the proposed reduction, both USPS and non-USPS FECA beneficiaries would have similar income from their FECA benefit package in comparison to their foregone FERS benefit.

In addition, under our simulation reduced FECA benefits were similar or less than FERS benefits across varying years of service.[28] However, as years of service increase, the gap between the two benefits widened. For example, we found that non-USPS beneficiaries whose total federal career would have spanned less than 10 years had a median reduced FECA benefit that was about 2 percent greater than the corresponding FERS benefit. In contrast, those non-USPS beneficiaries whose total federal career would have spanned 25-29 years had a median reduced FECA benefit that was 19 percent less than the corresponding FERS benefit. Similarly, USPS beneficiaries whose total federal career would have spanned less than 10 years had a median reduced FECA benefit that was about 13 percent greater than the corresponding FERS benefit. In contrast, USPS beneficiaries whose total federal career would have spanned 25 to 29 years had a median reduced FECA benefit that was 20 percent less than the corresponding FERS benefit.[29]

---

[28] In other words, under the proposed reduced FECA, based on our simulations, beneficiaries would have similar or less income in retirement than they would have had absent an injury.

[29] Because few people in our dataset had more than 25 years of federal service at the time of retirement, we do not capture those who would choose to work 30 or more years in the federal government before retiring.

Median Reduced FECA Benefit Packages Would Likely Be Less Than Median FERS Benefit Packages for Federal Annuitants with 30-Year Careers

Because FERS had only been in place for 26 years in 2010, our simulation did not capture the "mature" FERS benefit that an annuitant could accrue with more years of service. Consequently, it is likely that our analysis understates the potential FERS benefit when we consider 2010 benefit levels. As a result, we conducted a simulation of a "mature" FERS that was coupled with the assumption that individuals have 30-year federal careers. Based on this simulation, we found that the median current FECA benefit packages for non-USPS beneficiaries were on par or less than the median FERS benefit package—depending on the amount an individual contributes toward their TSP account for retirement. As shown on the right sides of figures 4 and 5, under the default scenario where there is no employee contribution and the employing agency contributes 1 percent to TSP, the median FECA benefit package is about 1 percent greater than the median FERS benefit package. However, under a scenario where each employee contributes 5 percent—and receives a 5 percent agency match—the median FECA benefit package is about 10 percent less than the median FERS benefit package. Similarly, our simulation showed that for USPS annuitants, the median FECA benefit package was about 13 percent greater than the median FERS benefit package under the 1 percent agency contribution scenario, and about 4 percent less than the median FERS benefit package under the 10 percent contribution scenario.

Figure 4: Median FECA and FERS Benefit Packages by Years of Service (Non-USPS)

Median total benefits (in dollars)

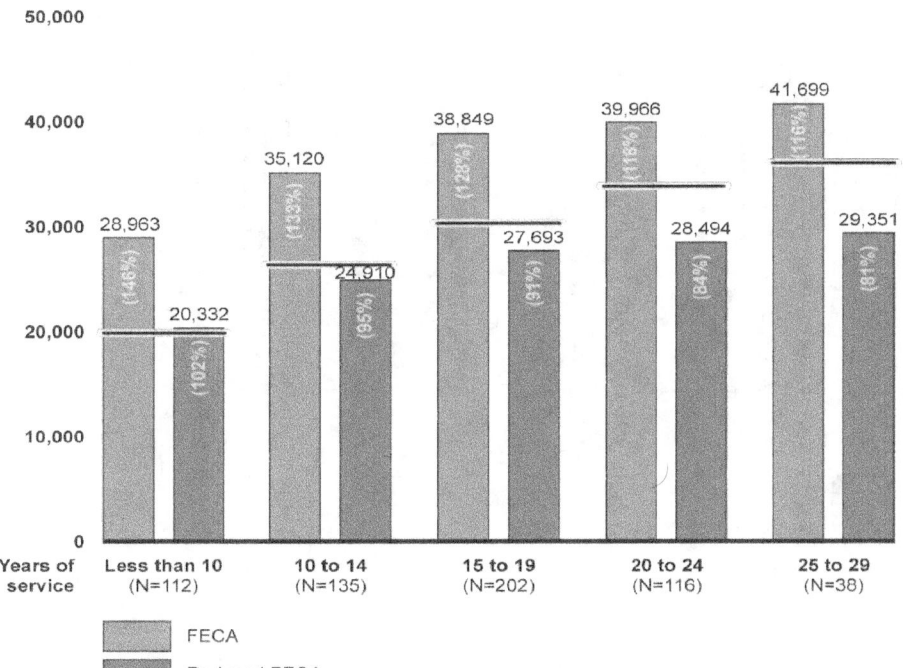
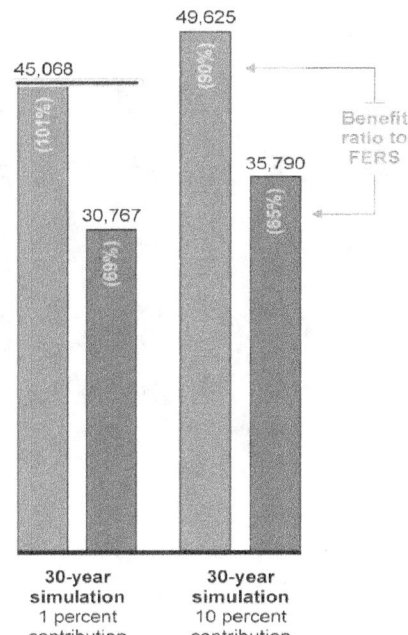

| Years of service | Less than 10 (N=112) | 10 to 14 (N=135) | 15 to 19 (N=202) | 20 to 24 (N=116) | 25 to 29 (N=38) | 30-year simulation 1 percent contribution | 30-year simulation 10 percent contribution |

Legend:
- FECA
- Reduced FECA
- FERS (current)

Source: GAO analysis of simulation results.

Figure 5: Median FECA and FERS Benefit Packages by Years of Service (USPS)

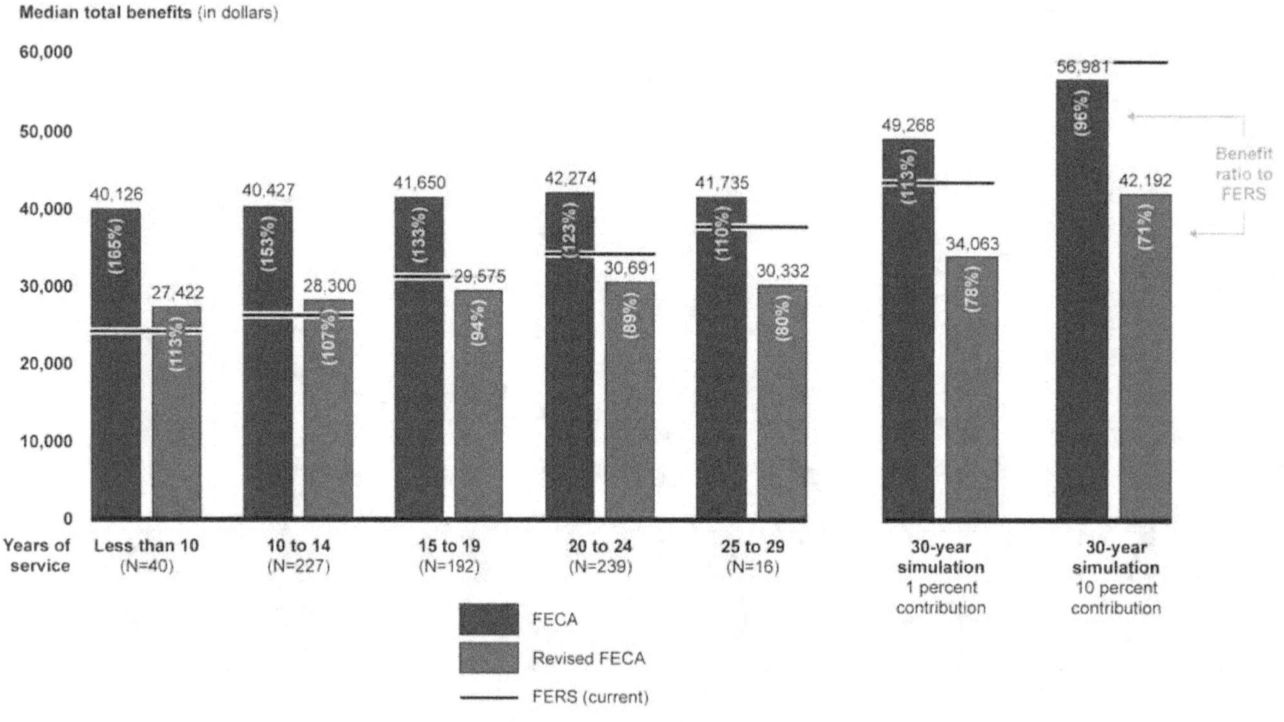

Median total benefits (in dollars)

| Years of service | Less than 10 (N=40) | 10 to 14 (N=227) | 15 to 19 (N=192) | 20 to 24 (N=239) | 25 to 29 (N=16) | 30-year simulation 1 percent contribution | 30-year simulation 10 percent contribution |

FECA

Revised FECA

FERS (current)

Source: GAO analysis of simulation results.

Our simulation also found that, for both non-USPS and USPS annuitants, the median reduced FECA benefit package under the proposed changes was less than the median FERS benefit package—regardless of the simulated contributions to TSP accounts. Specifically, under a scenario where there is no employee contribution—and a 1 percent contribution from the employing agency—the median reduced FECA benefit package is about 31 percent less than the median FERS benefit package for non-USPS annuitants and 22 percent less than the median FERS benefit package for USPS annuitants. Under a scenario where each employee contributes 5 percent—and receives a 5 percent agency match—the median reduced FECA benefit package is about 35 percent less than the FERS benefit package for non-USPS annuitants and about 29 percent less than the FERS benefit package for USPS annuitants.

Effects of Proposed FECA Revisions on Partial-disability Beneficiaries Depend on Post-Injury Earning Capacity and Employment Over Time

We found partial-disability beneficiaries to be fundamentally different from total-disability beneficiaries, as they receive reduced benefits based on their potential to be re-employed and have work earnings. However, there is limited information available about the overall population of partial-disability beneficiaries. They do not all find work and their participation in the workforce may change over time, and their individual experiences will determine how they would fare under the proposed revisions.

Total Income Comparisons for Partial-Disability Beneficiaries Under Single-Rate Proposals Depend on the Extent to Which Each Is Reemployed

Partial-disability beneficiaries in the case studies we examined fared differently under both FECA and the proposed revisions to pre-retirement compensation, depending on the extent to which they had work earnings in addition to their FECA benefits. To consider this larger context, we conducted total income comparisons for the partial-disability case studies we examined. We defined the post-injury total income comparison to be the sum of post-injury FECA benefits and any gross earnings from employment at the time of the LWEC decision, as a percentage of pre-injury gross income.[30]

Among the seven partial-disability case studies we examined, those beneficiaries with constructed earnings LWECs had post-injury total income comparisons that were substantially less than those with actual earnings LWECs. As shown in table 2, the beneficiaries in case studies 5-7 had constructed earnings LWECs and had post-injury total incomes that ranged from 29 to 65 percent of their pre-injury income under current FECA policy. This range was substantially lower than the total income comparisons for the beneficiaries in case studies 1-4 with actual earnings LWECs (77-96 percent). We found that by definition, at the time of their LWEC decision, those beneficiaries with constructed earnings LWECs earned less than the income OWCP used to calculate their LWECs. Consequently, their total income comparisons—FECA benefits plus earnings, as a percentage of pre-injury wages—are necessarily lower than those with actual earnings LWECs.

---

[30]This total income comparison is not the same as the wage replacement rate used in our prior analysis for total-disability beneficiaries. Total income includes FECA benefits and any gross earnings from work (not accounting for taxes). Post-injury earnings and FECA benefits are deflated to the time of injury to conduct a consistent comparison at a single point in time. For further details on the methodology, see enclosure I of GAO-13-143R.

Table 2: GAO Case Studies of Total Income Comparisons at Time of Loss of Wage Earning Capacity (LWEC) Decision

Case Study	Has a Dependent	Wages @ Injury[a]	Wages Post-Injury @ LWEC	Post-Injury Earning Capacity[b]	FECA Benefit @ Injury	Total Income Comparisons Under[c]		
						Current FECA Benefit Structure (pre-retirement)	Labor Proposal (pre-retirement compensation)	Senate Proposal (pre-retirement compensation)
1 - Returned to Agency	Yes	$52,684	$16,472	26%	$29,240	81.5%	77.8%	75.3%
2 - Returned to Agency	No	$28,691	$25,829	88%	$2,295	96.0%	96.4%	96.0%
3 - Private Sector Job	Yes	$75,724	$8,320	9%	$51,682	77.3%	72.7%	69.7%
4 - Private Sector Job	No	$38,675	$33,097	82%	$4,641	94.0%	94.6%	94.0%
5 - Constructed LWEC	Yes	$58,033	$5,383	26%	$32,208	64.5%	60.8%	58.3%
6 - Constructed LWEC	Yes	$35,082	$0	49%	$13,419	38.3%	35.7%	34.0%
7 - Constructed LWEC	No	$34,936	$0	56%	$10,248	29.3%	30.8%	29.3%

Source: GAO analysis of partial-disability case studies.

[a]The dollar amounts for wages and benefits are in nominal terms from the year of the injury or OWCP's LWEC decision; they are thus not comparable for each beneficiary or across beneficiaries. Dollars are standardized in the income comparisons and are thus comparable across beneficiaries (see enclosure I of GAO-13-143R for details on the methodology).

[b]Post-injury earning capacity represents OWCP's determination of a beneficiary's potential to earn wages. For instance, OWCP determined that the beneficiary in case study 1 had the potential to earn 26 percent of her wages at the time of injury.

[c]Total income comparisons represent each beneficiary's post-injury FECA benefits plus any gross earnings from employment at the time of the LWEC decision, as a percentage of his or her pre-injury gross income, under current FECA policy and the proposed revisions to pre-retirement benefits.

We also found that beneficiaries in our case studies were affected differently by the proposed revisions to pre-retirement benefits. As expected, the beneficiaries who did not have a dependent (case studies 2, 4, and 7) experienced either slight increases or no change in their post-injury total income comparisons under the proposed revisions to pre-retirement benefits. Under both proposals, the beneficiaries in our case studies who had a dependent (case studies 1, 3, 5, and 6) experienced declines in their post-injury total income comparisons.[31] However, these decreases in total income comparisons were relatively small compared to the impact of not having actual earnings. For instance, the beneficiary with a constructed earnings LWEC in case study 6 experienced declines in total income comparisons of about 3 to 4 percentage points between current FECA policy and the proposals. However, the beneficiary's total income comparisons under current FECA policy and the proposals were over 30 percentage points lower than those of the beneficiary in case study 3 who had the lowest total income comparisons of those beneficiaries with actual earnings LWECs.

Due to the importance of actual work earnings on partial-disability beneficiaries' situations, we have previously concluded that a snapshot of post-injury total income comparisons is insufficient to predict how beneficiaries fare over the remainder of their post-injury careers. Employment at the time of OWCP's LWEC decision does not necessarily imply stable employment over time, as beneficiaries can find, change, or lose jobs over time.

Effects of Proposals to Reduce FECA at Retirement Age Depend on Whether Partial-Disability Beneficiaries Remain on FECA or Elect OPM Retirement Benefits

We have also found that the proposals to reduce FECA benefits at retirement age would primarily affect those partial-disability beneficiaries who continue to receive FECA benefits past retirement age. As we reported in December 2012, among those partial-disability beneficiaries who stopped receiving FECA benefits in 2005-2011, 68 percent did so due to their election of OPM retirement or other benefits, such as Veterans Affairs disability benefits. At that time, Labor officials told us that because many variables affect retirement benefits, they cannot predict why partial-disability beneficiaries would potentially choose to retire instead of continuing to receive FECA benefits. Only 17 percent of partial-disability beneficiaries who stopped receiving FECA benefits were beneficiaries who died (i.e., received benefits from injury until death). These aggregate numbers do not track individual beneficiaries' decisions to elect retirement or to continue receiving FECA benefits past retirement age, but they suggest that there is a substantial percentage of partial-

---

[31]The proposals to compensate FECA beneficiaries at the single rate of 70 percent or 66-2/3 percent of wages at injury, regardless of the presence of dependents, would reduce pre-retirement FECA benefits for partial-disability beneficiaries with a dependent and would increase or have no effect on pre-retirement FECA benefits for those without a dependent, respectively.

disability beneficiaries that elects other benefits instead of FECA at some point post-injury.[32]

Since those beneficiaries who elect FERS retirement would not be affected by the proposed revisions to FECA compensation at retirement age, the overall effects of the proposals on partial-disability beneficiaries should be considered in the larger context of retirement options. To do so, in our December 2012 report, we used data from the seven partial-disability case studies to simulate and compare FERS and FECA benefits and to highlight various retirement options these partial-disability beneficiaries may face.[33] As shown in table 3, we found:

- The beneficiaries in case studies 2, 4, and 6 had potential FERS benefit packages that were higher than their FECA benefits under current policy and the proposed revision—they would likely not be affected by the proposed revision.

- The beneficiaries in case studies 1, 3, and 7 had potential FERS benefit packages that were lower than their FECA benefits under current policy and the proposed revision—they would likely face a reduction in FECA benefits in retirement under the proposed revision.

---

[32]While those beneficiaries who elect OPM retirement would not be affected by the proposals, they would receive lower retirement benefits than they would have had they never been injured, all else equal. Their federal careers were either shortened or they returned to federal employment at a reduced capacity—both of which would reduce their FERS annuities and Social Security benefits attributable to federal service.

[33]We compared potential FERS and FECA benefits for each beneficiary in the case studies at age 62—a common decision point for electing to retire and also consistent with our prior work—which measures what each beneficiary would actually receive though the beneficiaries were not actually retired. This comparison is thus not the same as the retirement counter-factual analysis conducted for total-disability beneficiaries that compared FECA benefits to retirement benefits if never injured. Although the proposed reduction would only go into effect once a beneficiary reaches full Social Security retirement age, we simulated the benefit reduction for all case studies, regardless of age. We did so to be consistent with our prior work, to present the comparison under each compensation rate, and to avoid imputing additional unknown years of service. Had we conducted the comparison at full Social Security retirement age, FECA benefits would have been larger due to additional cost of living adjustments and FERS benefits may have been larger due to additional years of service. We did not include Thrift Savings Plan (TSP) benefits or Social Security benefits attributable to non-federal service in the comparison because each beneficiary would have received those benefits whether they elected FERS retirement or chose to remain on FECA.

- The beneficiary in case study 5 had a potential FERS benefit package that was lower than his FECA benefits under current policy, but higher than his benefits under the proposed FECA reduction—he would likely face a reduction in FECA benefits in retirement under the proposed revision.

Table 3: GAO Case Studies: Benefits Comparisons at Retirement

Case Study	Has a Dependent	Wages @ Injury[a]	Wages Post-Injury @ LWEC	Post-Injury Earning Capacity[b]	Years of Federal Service[c]	Total Benefits Under Retirement:		
						Potential FERS Retirement Package	Current FECA Benefit Structure	Labor and Senate Proposals to Reduce FECA
1 - Returned to Agency	Yes	$52,684	$16,472	26%	14	$15,823	$34,554	$23,023
2 - Returned to Agency	No	$28,691	$25,829	88%	29	$24,410	$3,575	$2,678
3 - Private Sector Job	Yes	$75,724	$8,320	9%	17	$19,843	$75,023	$50,011
4 - Private Sector Job	No	$38,675	$33,097	82%	17	$13,513	$6,318	$4,758
5 - Constructed LWEC	Yes	$58,033	$5,383	26%	23	$25,518	$38,077	$25,376
6 - Constructed LWEC	Yes	$35,082	$0	49%	20	$17,132	$16,536	$11,011
7 - Constructed LWEC	No	$34,936	$0	56%	6	$7,905	$15,808	$11,830

Source: GAO analysis of partial-disability case studies.

[a]The dollar amounts for wages are in nominal terms from the year of the injury or OWCP's LWEC decision; they are thus not comparable for each beneficiary or across beneficiaries. Benefit comparison dollars are in nominal terms, but as of the same year for each individual; FERS and FECA benefits are thus comparable for each beneficiary, but not across beneficiaries (see enclosure I of GAO-13-143R for details on the methodology).

[b]Post-injury earning capacity represents OWCP's determination of a beneficiary's potential to earn wages. For instance, OWCP determined that the beneficiary in case study 1 had the potential to earn 26 percent of her wages at the time of injury.

[c]Years of federal service includes any additional years of service added to advance beneficiaries who were not yet 62 to age 62—the point of benefit comparison. See enclosure I of GAO-13-143R for additional details on the methodology.

[d]Total benefits in retirement compares the potential FERS retirement package if a beneficiary elects OPM retirement, FECA benefits under current FECA policy, and FECA benefits under the Labor and Senate proposals. Social Security benefits not attributable to federal service and TSP benefits were not included in the analysis because they cancel out on both sides of the comparison; whatever TSP balance and Social Security benefits attributable to non-federal employment a beneficiary had accrued would be theirs whether they elected FECA benefits or FERS retirement.

Based on our prior work, we have concluded that the differences in retirement options that individual beneficiaries face stem from two key factors: (1) OWCP's determination of their earning capacities, and (2) their total years of federal service. Partial-disability beneficiaries with greater potential for earnings from work receive relatively lower FECA benefits to account for their relatively lower loss of wage earning capacity, all else equal. In table 2, beneficiaries with:

- low earning capacities post-injury (case studies 1, 3, and 5) had FECA benefits that were more favorable than FERS benefits;

- high earning capacities post-injury (case studies 2 and 4) had FECA benefits that were less favorable than FERS benefits; and

- mid-range earning capacities post-injury (case studies 6 and 7) had FECA benefits whose favorability depended on their total years of federal service. Fewer years of federal service resulted in a lower FERS annuity and lower Social Security benefits attributable to federal service, all else equal.

We have also found that partial-disability beneficiaries who choose to remain on FECA past retirement age currently face lower FECA benefits in retirement as compared with total-disability beneficiaries, and would experience a reduction in benefits under the proposals. Partial-disability beneficiaries receive FECA benefits that are lower than those of otherwise identical total-disability beneficiaries to account for their potential for work earnings. As long as they work, their income is comprised of their earnings and their FECA benefits. However, once they choose to retire, partial-disability beneficiaries who choose to stay on FECA likely no longer have any work earnings and are not eligible to simultaneously receive their FERS annuity.[34] Thus, we found that because of the way FECA benefits are currently calculated, such partial-disability beneficiaries may have less income in retirement than otherwise identical total-disability beneficiaries, and the proposals would reduce benefits in retirement without differentiating between partial and total-

[34]Eligible total and partial-disability FECA beneficiaries may elect OPM retirement, such as under FERS, in lieu of FECA benefits.

disability beneficiaries.[35] The proposed reduction may serve as a long-term incentive for partial-disability beneficiaries to return to work,[36] particularly because their initial FECA benefits are lower than those of total-disability beneficiaries.

In conclusion, FECA continues to play a vital role in providing compensation to federal employees who are unable to work because of injuries sustained while performing their federal duties and FECA benefits generally serve as the exclusive remedy for being injured on the job. Our simulations of the potential effects of proposed changes to FECA benefit levels incorporated the kinds of approaches used in the literature on assessing benefit adequacy for workers' compensation programs, such as taking account of missed career growth. More specifically, we assessed the proposed changes by simulating the level of take-home pay or retirement benefits FECA beneficiaries would have received if they had not been injured, which provides a realistic basis for assessing how beneficiaries may be affected. However, we did not recommend any particular level of benefit adequacy. As policymakers assess proposed changes to FECA benefit levels, they will implicitly be making decisions about what constitutes an adequate level of benefits for FECA beneficiaries before and after they reach retirement age. While our analyses focused on how the median FECA beneficiary might be affected by proposed changes, it also highlighted how potential effects may vary for different subpopulations of beneficiaries, which can assist policymakers as they consider such changes to the FECA program.

This concludes my statement and I would be happy to answer any questions.

---

[35]Those partial-disability beneficiaries who were re-employed in non-federal jobs (e.g., in the private sector) can remain on FECA and receive any non-federal retirement benefits they may have accrued; similarly, those who were re-employed in federal jobs and remain on FECA in retirement may receive greater TSP benefits from any additional contributions during their re-employment.

[36]For example, by returning to work, partial-disability beneficiaries would be able to increase their potential FERS benefits with additional years of federal service and contributions to TSP, or obtain non-federal retirement benefits through other employment that could supplement their lower FERS or FECA benefits (depending on their retirement elections). Not all partial-disability beneficiaries return to work.

Contacts and Staff Acknowledgments

For further information regarding this testimony, please contact Andrew Sherrill at (202) 512-7215 or sherrilla@gao.gov. Contact points for our Offices of Congressional Relations and Public Affairs may be found on the last page of this statement. Individuals who made key contributions to this testimony include: Nagla'a El-Hodiri, Assistant Director; James Bennett, Jessica Botsford, Sherwin Chapman, Michael J. Collins, Melinda Cordero, Holly Dye, Michael Kniss, Gene Kuehneman, Kathy Leslie, James Rebbe, Jeff Tessin, Walter Vance, and Rebecca Woiwode.